# Peripheral Neuropathy Diet Cookbook For Beginners

## Nerve-Friendly Antidepressant Recipes for Restoring Sensation, Strengthening Weakness, and Managing Pain

Rose V Allen

## About the Author

In the bustling metropolis of New York City, Rose V. Allen, a dedicated nutritionist and culinary enthusiast, discovered her calling in the kitchen. Armed with a degree in nutrition, Rose graduated with second-class honours from Harvard State University, solidifying her expertise in the field. Drawing from her extensive educational background and fueled by a passion for helping others, she embarked on a journey to create recipes that not only delighted the palate but also served as potent remedies. With years of hands-on experience in the realm of nutrition, Rose understood the intricate connection between food and health. Having personally grappled with the challenges of peripheral neuropathy, she was uniquely positioned to offer solutions rooted in both science and compassion. Meticulously crafting each recipe in her cookbook, Rose infused them with the specific aim of alleviating symptoms and promoting healing. As a proud citizen of the United States, Rose's cookbook, "Peripheral Neuropathy Diet Cookbook for Beginners," stands as a testament to her unwavering commitment to helping others find relief and renewal through the transformative power of food.

# TABLE OF CONTENT

## INTRODUCTION

Embark on a voyage of health and vitality with the help of therapeutic nutrients and mouth-watering flavors in the Peripheral Neuropathy Diet Cookbook. Join me on a quest—a quest for flavor, better health, and personal growth.

Let me introduce you to Sarah. Sarah was a free spirit who had always thrived on the dance floor and the woods. But then, all of a sudden, her feet started to tingle, and it spread like a quiet thief taking her feelings. Pain, weakness, and aggravation replaced the tingling at some point. An ailment that threatened to diminish Sarah's life's vitality was peripheral neuropathy, which she was diagnosed with.

Peripheral neuropathy affects many people and may have a significant influence on their day-to-day life, just like Sarah. Tingling, numbness, muscular weakness, or constant discomfort are all symptoms that could make the obstacles appear insurmountable. But in the darkness of doubt, there's a light of hope—a road lit by the power of nourishment.

As Sarah navigated her path, she found the transformational power of food. With each meticulously constructed meal, she experienced relief from her symptoms, a fresh feeling of vitality, and a deeper understanding of the relationship between what she ate and how she felt. And so, the concept for this cookbook was born—not simply as a compilation of dishes, but as a guiding light for anyone seeking peace and support on their neuropathy journey.

Within these pages, you'll discover more than simply materials and directions; you'll find empowerment, inspiration, and the promise of a better future.

But this cookbook isn't only for individuals afflicted with peripheral neuropathy. It's for caretakers supporting their loved ones, for health enthusiasts trying to enhance their well-being, and for anybody willing to embrace the healing power of food.

So, when you go on this gastronomic journey, realize that you're not alone. Together, we'll explore the delightful junction of taste and health, one dish at a time. Welcome to the Peripheral Neuropathy Diet Cookbook—where food meets repair, and every mouthful gets us closer to a life lived to its utmost potential.

# CHAPTER ONE

## Understanding Peripheral Neuropathy: Causes, Symptoms, and Management

Imagine strolling down a sandy beach, feeling the warmth of the sun on your skin and the gentle grains under your feet. Now, picture that feeling progressively slipping away, replaced by an uncomfortable numbness, tingling, or even pain. This is the reality for millions of persons living with peripheral neuropathy—a disorder that may significantly disrupt everyday life.

But what precisely is peripheral neuropathy, and how does it impact us? Let's dig into the subtleties of this ailment, investigating its origins, symptoms, and measures for successful care.

At its heart, peripheral neuropathy is a complicated condition defined by damage to the peripheral nerves—the extensive network that links the brain and spinal cord to the rest of the body. This damage may come from several reasons, including:

- Diabetes: Elevated blood sugar levels over time may cause nerve damage, especially in the limbs.
- Trauma: Injuries, accidents, or procedures may lead to nerve compression or injury.
- Autoimmune Disorders: Conditions such as lupus, rheumatoid arthritis, and Guillain-Barré syndrome may generate immune responses that attack the neurological system.
- Infections: Viral or bacterial infections, such as shingles or Lyme disease, may disrupt nerve function.

- Toxins: Exposure to certain chemicals, drugs, or environmental toxins may lead to nerve injury.

- Nutritional Deficiencies: Inadequate consumption of vital nutrients like vitamin B12 or folate might affect neuron health.

Regardless of the underlying etiology, the symptoms of peripheral neuropathy might vary greatly from person to person. Some people may experience:

- Numbness or tingling generally begins in the hands or feet and expands gradually.

- Burning or shooting pain, which may exacerbate at night or with movement.

- Muscle weakness, resulting in difficulties with actions like holding items or walking.

- Sensitivity to touch or temperature changes.

**Coordination and balance difficulties, increase the risk of falls.**

Living with these symptoms might be tough, but there is hope. Effective care of peripheral neuropathy frequently entails a multimodal strategy, treating both the underlying cause and the symptoms itself. Some major tactics include:

- Controlling Blood Sugar Levels: For persons with diabetes, keeping stable blood glucose levels is critical for avoiding additional nerve damage.
- Drugs: Certain drugs, such as anticonvulsants, antidepressants, or pain relievers, may help lessen neuropathic pain.

- Physical Therapy: Targeted exercises may improve strength, flexibility, and balance, lowering the risk of falls and boosting overall quality of life.

- Nerve-Specific Supplements: Nutritional supplements including alpha-lipoic acid, acetyl-L-carnitine, and certain vitamins may promote nerve health and function.

- Lifestyle Modifications: Making good lifestyle choices, such as stopping smoking, reducing alcohol use, and keeping a balanced diet, may increase general well-being.

As we go further into the pages of this cookbook, we'll examine how diet plays a crucial part in controlling peripheral neuropathy symptoms. By filling our bodies with healthy meals rich in vitamins, minerals, antioxidants, and anti-inflammatory chemicals, we can maintain nerve health and decrease pain.

So, whether you're battling with peripheral neuropathy yourself or looking to help a loved one on their journey, recognizing the subtleties of this ailment is the first step toward appropriate care. Together, let's empower ourselves with knowledge, resilience, and the unflinching hope that better days are ahead.

# CHAPTER TWO

## The Role of Nutrition in Managing Peripheral Neuropathy

Picture this: Your body is a highly tuned machine, with each nutrient functioning as a critical cog in the complicated mechanics of health. Now, suppose some of these vital components are missing, causing the gears to grind and falter. This comparison brilliantly highlights the significant influence that diet can have on controlling peripheral neuropathy—a disease where supporting our bodies with the correct foods becomes not simply a choice, but a cornerstone of wellbeing.

Peripheral neuropathy, with its multitude of symptoms ranging from numbness and tingling to excruciating pain and weakness, poses a unique set of issues.

But within the intricacies of this situation, there emerges a tremendous ally: the food we consume. Let's look into the function of diet in controlling peripheral neuropathy and unlocking the possibility of healing from within.

At its core, nutrition acts as the fuel that fuels our bodies, giving the basic elements required for cellular repair, regeneration, and function. For patients suffering from peripheral neuropathy, maximizing this fuel becomes crucial, since specific nutrients play a vital role in sustaining nerve health and alleviating symptoms.

**Key nutrients for controlling peripheral neuropathy include:**

- B Vitamins: The B-complex vitamins—particularly B1 (thiamine), B6 (pyridoxine), B12 (cobalamin), and folate—are needed for nerve function and repair. Deficiencies in these vitamins have been related to neuropathic symptoms, making their replenishment a cornerstone of therapy.

- Antioxidants: Free radicals—unstable chemicals that may harm cells and tissues—are linked to nerve injury and inflammation associated with peripheral neuropathy. Antioxidants like vitamins C and E, as well as chemicals found in colored fruits and vegetables, help neutralize these toxic molecules, affording protection to sensitive nerve fibers.

- Omega-3 Fatty Acids: Found abundantly in fatty fish, flaxseeds, and walnuts, omega-3 fatty acids exhibit significant anti-inflammatory qualities, which may help ease pain and reduce nerve inflammation in persons with peripheral neuropathy.

- Minerals: Essential minerals such as magnesium, calcium, and zinc play essential roles in nerve signaling, muscular function, and general nervous system health. Ensuring proper intake of these minerals via food or supplementation is crucial for treating neuropathic symptoms.

- Plant molecules: Phytochemicals—bioactive molecules present in plant foods—exert protective effects on nerve cells, lowering oxidative stress and inflammation. Incorporating a range of colored fruits, vegetables, herbs, and spices into your diet may offer a wide assortment of phytonutrients to promote nerve health.

By harnessing the power of these nutrients via a balanced and diverse diet, persons with peripheral neuropathy may fuel their bodies from the inside out, fostering healing, resilience, and vigor. But the path doesn't stop with merely knowing which foods to eat—it also entails mindful eating behaviors, portion management, and a dedication to consistency and sustainability.

As we travel through the pages of this cookbook, we'll discover tasty meals and culinary delights meant to enhance nerve health and decrease neuropathic symptoms. From nutrient-packed smoothies to savory main courses and luscious desserts, each recipe is deliberately prepared to feed your body and excite your taste buds, illustrating that controlling peripheral neuropathy can be both a journey of recovery and a celebration of gastronomic joy.

So, join us as we start on this gourmet trip, where the transformational power of food meets the tenacity of the human spirit. Together, let's relish the pleasures of healing and accept the nurturing embrace of nutrition in controlling peripheral neuropathy.

## How This Cookbook Can Help You

Welcome to a culinary adventure unlike any other—a voyage that transcends the world of ordinary recipes and ingredients to provide you with a lifeline in the face of peripheral neuropathy. As you hold this cookbook in your hands, you're not only carrying a selection of wonderful foods; you're holding a roadmap to recovering your energy, one mouthful at a time. But how precisely might this cookbook assist you on your road toward treating peripheral neuropathy and regaining the pleasure of eating? Let's explore.

- Tailored Recipes for Nerve Health: Within these pages, you'll discover a treasure trove of recipes precisely developed to feed your nerves and calm your symptoms. From nutrient-dense smoothies to warm soups, vivid salads, and fulfilling main courses, each recipe is developed with your well-being in mind, containing important elements proven to improve nerve function and minimize neuropathic symptoms.

- Culinary Innovation Meets Scientific Rigor: Behind every dish lies a mix of culinary innovation and scientific rigor. Drawing inspiration from the latest studies on nutrition and neuropathy treatment, our team of specialists has carefully handpicked a range of recipes that not only tempt the taste senses but also give practical advantages to your nervous system. With each ingredient picked carefully and each cooking process optimized for optimum nutrient retention, you can trust that every meal takes you closer to optimal health.

- Empowerment Through Education: This cookbook is more than simply a collection of recipes—it's a complete resource that empowers you with the information and awareness required to take charge of your health. Throughout these pages, you'll discover insights on the importance of nutrition in managing peripheral neuropathy, practical ideas for meal planning and preparation, and help in making educated food choices to promote your well-being. Armed with this information, you'll not only fuel your body but also build a deeper relationship with the food you consume and the influence it has on your health.

- Practical Solutions for Real-Life Challenges: We recognize that controlling peripheral neuropathy comes with its own set of obstacles, from negotiating dietary restrictions to finding the time and energy to make healthful meals. That's why this cookbook is full of practical answers to help you overcome these challenges and adopt nerve-friendly food into your everyday life. Whether you're a rookie in the kitchen or a seasoned cook, you'll discover recipes and ideas adapted to your requirements, making healthy eating both accessible and pleasurable.

- Community and Support: Last but not least, this cookbook is a monument to the power of community and support in the path toward health and recovery.

Within these pages, you'll discover tales of perseverance, encouragement from other travelers on the neuropathy route, and ways to connect with others suffering similar issues. Whether you're seeking help, inspiration, or just a listening ear, you'll discover a supportive community willing to walk with you every step of the journey.

So, as you begin on this gastronomic journey, know that you're not alone. With this cookbook as your guide, you have all you need to fuel your body, ease your symptoms, and recapture your energy. Together, let's embrace the transformational power of food and go on a journey of healing, one delicious meal at a time.

**Exploring Key Nutrients for Nerve Health**

In the rich tapestry of human health, few threads are more crucial than the nutrients that fuel our nerves—the fragile fibers that comprise the sophisticated communication network connecting our brains to every area of our body. As we dive into the area of treating peripheral neuropathy, knowing these important nutrients becomes not simply a matter of curiosity, but a cornerstone of healing and resilience.

Let's begin on a voyage of inquiry, revealing the nutrients that possess the capacity to enhance nerve health, alleviate neuropathic symptoms, and kindle the flame of energy inside us.

- B Vitamins: The backbone of nerve health, B vitamins play a major role in sustaining the integrity of our neural system. Among them, vitamin B12 stands out as a superhero, required for nerve cell function and the development of myelin—the protective coating that surrounds nerve fibers. Deficiencies in B12, as well as other B vitamins including thiamine (B1) and pyridoxine (B6), have been associated with neuropathic symptoms such as tingling, numbness, and weakness. Incorporating B vitamin-rich foods like lean meats, fish, eggs, dairy products, leafy greens, and fortified cereals into your diet will assist promote healthy nerve function and vitality.

- Antioxidants: In the struggle against oxidative stress—a characteristic of peripheral neuropathy—antioxidants emerge as our friends, employing their protective qualities to shield nerve cells from injury. Vitamins C and E, together with substances like beta-carotene and selenium, neutralize damaging free radicals, decreasing inflammation and avoiding cellular damage. Colorful fruits and vegetables, nuts, seeds, and whole grains are great sources of antioxidants, delivering a robust defense against neuropathic symptoms.

- Omega-3 Fatty Acids: Like soothing balm for inflamed nerves, omega-3 fatty acids exhibit exceptional anti-inflammatory characteristics that may help reduce neuropathic pain and suffering. Found abundantly in fatty fish like salmon, mackerel, and sardines, as well as in plant-based sources like flaxseeds, chia seeds, and walnuts, these essential fatty acids provide a natural cure for relaxing stressed nerves and improving general well-being.

- Minerals: Magnesium, calcium, and potassium—these minerals aren't simply needed for healthy bones and muscles; they're also crucial actors in the delicate dance of nerve transmission and function. Magnesium, in particular, works as a natural muscle relaxant, relieving tension and cramping typically associated with peripheral neuropathy. Leafy greens, nuts, seeds, legumes, and whole grains are good suppliers of these nerve-nourishing minerals, giving a delectable road to pain alleviation and relaxation.

- Alpha-Lipoic Acid: As a potent antioxidant and nerve-regenerating agent, alpha-lipoic acid shows tremendous promise in the care of peripheral neuropathy. This substance not only scavenges free radicals and lowers inflammation but also improves glucose absorption in nerve cells, encouraging energy generation and neuron healing. Sources of alpha-lipoic acid include spinach, broccoli, tomatoes, and organ meats, as well as supplements available in capsule or tablet form.

As we immerse ourselves in the world of these critical nutrients for nerve health, let us remember that the route to recovery starts with the choices we make each day—the meals we pick, the tastes we relish, and the sustenance we offer to our bodies and spirits. Together, let's embrace the transformational power of nutrition and begin on a journey toward bright health and vitality, one nutrient-rich food at a time.

## Understanding the Impact of Diet on Peripheral Neuropathy Symptoms

Imagine your body as a perfectly tuned instrument, each note resonating with the foods you consume—a symphony of tastes and nutrients orchestrating your health and well-being. Now, imagine the enormous influence that nutrition may have on the complicated dance of peripheral neuropathy symptoms—the tingling, numbness, pain, and weakness that characterize this disorder. In this investigation, we explore the complicated connection between nutrition and peripheral neuropathy symptoms, exposing the transformational potential of feeding your body from the inside.

Peripheral neuropathy is a complicated disorder defined by damage to the peripheral nerves—the extensive network that links your brain and spinal cord to the rest of your body. While the underlying reasons for neuropathy may vary—from diabetes and autoimmune illnesses to infections and toxin exposure—the function of nutrition in treating its symptoms remains apparent.

So, how does nutrition affect peripheral neuropathy symptoms? Let's go into the nuances:

- Blood Sugar Control: For persons with diabetes—a prevalent underlying cause of neuropathy—maintaining stable blood sugar levels is crucial. Fluctuations in blood glucose may aggravate nerve injury and increase neuropathic symptoms. By adopting a balanced diet rich in complex carbs, fiber, lean proteins, and healthy fats, you may help manage blood sugar levels and limit the risk of nerve damage.

- Inflammation Management: Inflammation sits at the core of many chronic health problems, including peripheral neuropathy. Certain dietary choices—such as processed meals, sugary snacks, and unhealthy fats—can fuel inflammation, aggravating neuropathic pain and suffering. Conversely, a diet rich in anti-inflammatory foods—such as fruits, vegetables, whole grains, and omega-3 fatty acids—can help reduce inflammation and ease neuropathic symptoms.

- Nerve-Nourishing Nutrients: Just as a garden flourishes with the appropriate combination of nutrients, so too can your nerves flourish when fed with the right foods. Nutrients including vitamins B12, B6, and E, as well as alpha-lipoic acid, magnesium, and antioxidants, play key roles in sustaining nerve health and function. By integrating nutrient-dense foods into your diet—such as leafy greens, lean meats, nuts, seeds, and colorful fruits and vegetables—you offer your nerves the building blocks they need to grow.

- Weight Management: Excess weight may worsen neuropathic symptoms, putting more strain on nerves and limiting circulation. Adopting a balanced diet and indulging in regular physical exercise may help maintain a healthy weight, minimizing the pressure on your nerves and increasing overall well-being.

- Gut Health: Emerging research reveals a close relationship between gut health and brain function, with alterations in gut microbiota associated with numerous neurological illnesses, including neuropathy. By fueling your gut with a varied selection of fiber-rich meals, fermented foods, and prebiotics, you maintain a healthy microbiota and promote optimum nerve health.

As you negotiate the complexity of treating peripheral neuropathy, remember that the foods you pick may either feed inflammation and increase symptoms or nourish your nerves and encourage recovery. By adopting a diet rich in nutrient-dense, anti-inflammatory foods, you empower yourself to take charge of your health and go on a road toward symptom alleviation and vitality.

Together, let's harness the transforming power of nutrition and unleash the possibility of healing from within. As you relish the sensations of food and vigor, may each meal bring you closer to a life lived completely and joyously, despite the obstacles of peripheral neuropathy.

## Stocking Your Pantry: Essential Ingredients for Nerve-Nourishing Meals

Welcome to the heart of your culinary sanctuary—the pantry. Here, between shelves stacked with jars and sacks, lies the cornerstone of your path toward nerve health and vitality. As you begin on the road of controlling peripheral neuropathy via diet, filling your pantry with important ingredients becomes not just a job, but a holy ritual—a physical representation of your devotion to feeding your body from the inside.

But what precisely are these vital ingredients—the building blocks of nerve-nourishing meals? Let's explore the riches that await inside your pantry, each one offering the promise of healing, resilience, and rebirth.

- Whole Grains: At the cornerstone of every healthful pantry lies an assortment of whole grains—ancient treasures rich in fiber, vitamins, minerals, and complex carbs. From robust oats and nutty quinoa to aromatic brown rice and adaptable whole wheat pasta, these grains provide the backbone of nerve-nourishing meals, giving lasting energy and important nutrients to drive your path toward vitality.

- Legumes: Bursting with plant-based protein, fiber, and an assortment of vitamins and minerals, legumes are a pantry essential for nerve health and well-being. Whether you favor creamy lentils, string beans, or delicate chickpeas, these modest legumes provide a flexible canvas for producing healthy soups, stews, salads, and dips, all while keeping stable blood sugar levels and supporting digestive health.

- Nuts and Seeds: Nature's nutrient-rich gems, nuts, and seeds are filled with heart-healthy fats, protein, fiber, and an assortment of vitamins and minerals important for nerve function and repair. From crunchy almonds and creamy cashews to omega-3-rich flaxseeds and chia seeds, these culinary treasures bring texture, taste, and nutritional punch to your meals, snacks, and baked products.

- Healthy Oils: When it comes to cooking and decorating your culinary masterpieces, selecting healthy oils may make all the difference in supporting nerve health and lowering inflammation. Extra-virgin olive oil, rich in monounsaturated fats and antioxidants, is a tasty option for sautéing and drizzling, while avocado oil and coconut oil provide flexibility and stability at high temperatures.

- Herbs & Spices: Elevate your cuisine from ordinary to spectacular with the bright tastes and therapeutic capabilities of herbs and spices. From aromatic basil and zesty ginger to warming cinnamon and fragrant turmeric, these culinary powerhouses not only tempt the taste senses but also claim anti-inflammatory, antioxidant, and neuroprotective capabilities, increasing both the flavor and therapeutic value of your meals.

- Colorful Fruits and Vegetables: No pantry is complete without an array of colorful fruits and vegetables—the brilliant gems of nature's wealth. Rich in vitamins, minerals, antioxidants, and phytonutrients, these plant-based jewels provide a rainbow of tastes and textures to inspire your culinary creativity, while supporting nerve health, lowering inflammation, and promoting overall well-being.

As you fill your pantry with these basic components, remember that you're not merely filling shelves; you're nurturing a sanctuary of healing and nourishment—a place where every item offers the promise of life and rebirth. So, embrace the trip, relish the flavors, and allow the nurturing embrace of your pantry to lead you toward a life lived completely and cheerfully, despite the limitations of peripheral neuropathy.

# CHAPTER THREE

**Breakfasts to Jumpstart Your Day**

**Warm Quinoa Breakfast dish**

This substantial breakfast dish is filled with protein and fiber to keep you energetic throughout the morning.

Preparation Time: 5 minutes

Cooking Time: 20 minutes

Total Time: 25 minutes

Serving Size: 2

**Ingredients:**

- 1 cup quinoa, washed
- 2 cups almond milk
- 1 tablespoon honey
- 1/2 teaspoon cinnamon
- 1/4 cup sliced almonds
- Fresh berries for topping

**Method of Preparation:**

1. In a saucepan, mix quinoa and almond milk. Bring to a boil, then decrease heat and simmer for 15-20 minutes until quinoa is cooked.

2. Stir in honey and cinnamon.

3. Divide quinoa into bowls and top with sliced almonds and fresh berries.

**Banana Nut Oatmeal**

Creamy oatmeal with bananas and almonds gives a warm and healthy start to your day.

Preparation Time: 5 minutes

Cooking Time: 10 minutes

Total Time: 15 minutes

Serving Size: 2

**Ingredients**:

- 1 cup rolled oats
- 2 cups water
- 1 ripe banana, mashed

- 2 teaspoons chopped walnuts

- 1 tablespoon maple syrup

**Method of Preparation:**

1. In a saucepan, bring water to a boil. Stir in rolled oats and lower heat to medium-low. Cook for 5-7 minutes, stirring periodically, until oats are cooked.

2. Stir in mashed banana and chopped walnuts.

3. Drizzle with maple syrup before serving.

**Avocado Toast with Poached Egg**

Creamy avocado coupled with a flawlessly poached egg over whole grain bread makes for a pleasant and healthy meal or brunch.

Preparation Time: 10 minutes

Cooking Time: 5 minutes

Total Time: 15 minutes

Serving Size: 2

**Ingredients:**

- 2 slices whole grain bread
- 1 ripe avocado, mashed
- 2 eggs
- Salt and pepper to taste
- Red pepper flakes (optional)

**Method of Preparation:**

1. Toast the whole grain bread slices till golden brown.
2. Spread mashed avocado evenly over the toasted bread pieces.

3. In a saucepan, bring water to a low simmer. Crack eggs, one at a time, into a small dish and delicately slip them into the heating water. Poach eggs for 3-4 minutes until whites are set but yolks are still liquid.

4. Using a slotted spoon, gently take poached eggs from the water and lay them on top of the avocado toast.

5. Season with salt, pepper, and red pepper flakes if preferred. Serve immediately.

**Berry Smoothie Bowl**

A refreshing and antioxidant-rich smoothie bowl topped with fresh berries and crunchy granola is the ideal way to start your day on a healthy note.

Preparation Time: 5 minutes

Total Time: 5 minutes

Serving Size: 2

**Ingredients:**

- 1 cup mixed berries (strawberries, blueberries, raspberries)
- 1 ripe banana
- 1/2 cup Greek yogurt
- 1/4 cup almond milk
- 2 tablespoons honey or maple syrup
- Granola, sliced almonds, and more berries for topping

**Method of Preparation:**

1. In a blender, combine mixed berries, banana, Greek yogurt, almond milk, and honey or maple syrup. Blend until smooth and creamy.

2. Pour the smoothie into bowls and top with granola, sliced almonds, and more berries.

3. Serve immediately and enjoy with a spoon!

**Spinach and Mushroom Frittata**

This protein-packed frittata laden with spinach and mushrooms is excellent for a leisurely weekend brunch or a quick weekday breakfast.

Preparation Time: 10 minutes

Cooking Time: 20 minutes

Total Time: 30 minutes

Serving Size: 4

**Ingredients**

- 6 big eggs

- 1/4 cup milk

- 1 tablespoon olive oil

- 2 cups fresh spinach leaves

- 1 cup sliced mushrooms

- 1/2 onion, diced

- Salt and pepper to taste

- 1/4 cup shredded cheese (optional)

**Method of Preparation:**

1. Preheat the oven to 350°F (175°C).

2. In a bowl, mix eggs and milk. Season with salt and pepper.

3. Heat olive oil to a simmer in an oven-proof skillet over medium heat. Add chopped onion and sliced mushrooms, and heat until softened, approximately 5 minutes.

4. Add fresh spinach leaves to the pan and simmer until wilted.

5. Spread the egg mixture over the veggies in the skillet. Sauté for 2-3 minutes until the outer edges start to set.

6. Sprinkle shredded cheese over the top, if using.

7. Transfer the pan to the preheated oven and bake for 10-12 minutes, until the frittata is set and slightly browned on top.

8. Remove from the oven and let cool for a few minutes before slicing. Serve warm.

# CHAPTER FOUR

**Nourishing Lunch Ideas**

**Salad with Grilled Salmon and Avocado**

This colorful salad is a healthy and filling lunch choice thanks to the grilled salmon, creamy avocado, and a variety of fresh veggies.

Preparations Time: 10 minutes .

Cooking Time: 10 minutes

Total Time: 20 minutes

Serving Size: 2

**Ingredients**

- fillets of salmon, two
- Toss with salt and pepper.
- 1 sliced avocado 4 cups of mixed greens (lettuce, arugula, and spinach)
- 1 cup cherry tomatoes, halved
- 1/4 red onion, thinly sliced
- 2 tablespoons olive oil

- 1 tablespoon balsamic vinegar

- 1 teaspoon Dijon mustard

**Method of Preparation:**

1. Season salmon fillets with salt and pepper. Grill for 4-5 minutes on each side, until cooked through.

2. In a large bowl, add mixed greens, sliced avocado, cherry tomatoes, and thinly sliced red onion.

3. In a small bowl, mix olive oil, balsamic vinegar, and Dijon mustard to create the dressing.

4. Spread the dressing throughout the salad and stir to coat completely.

5. Divide the salad across two dishes and top each with a grilled salmon fillet.

6. Serve immediately and enjoy this healthful and tasty salad.

**Turkey and Veggie Wrap with Hummus**

This easy-to-make wrap is loaded with lean turkey, crisp veggies, and creamy hummus, making it a delightful and filling lunch alternative.

Preparation Time: 10 minutes

Total Time: 10 minutes

Serving Size: 2

**Ingredients**

- 2 big whole-wheat tortillas
- 4 tablespoons hummus
- 8 slices deli turkey
- 1/2 cucumber, thinly sliced
- 1/2 red bell pepper, thinly sliced
- Handful of spinach leaves
- Toss with salt and pepper.

## Method of Preparation

1. Lay out the whole wheat tortillas on a clean surface.

2. Spread 2 tablespoons of hummus equally over each tortilla.

3. Layer 4 slices of deli turkey on each tortilla, followed by cucumber slices, red bell pepper slices, and spinach leaves.

4. Season with salt and pepper to taste.

5. Roll up the wraps securely, tucking in the sides as you go.

6. Slice each wrap in half diagonally and serve immediately.

## Lentil Soup with Spinach and Tomatoes

This hearty lentil soup is full of healthful veggies and protein-packed lentils, making it a cozy and delicious dish for lunch or supper.

Takes around ten minutes to prepare.

Cooking Time: 30 minutes

Total Time: 40 minutes

Serving Size: 4

**Ingredients:**

- 1 cup dry green lentils, washed
- 1 tablespoon olive oil
- 1 onion, diced 2 carrots, diced
- 2 celery stalks, chopped
- 3 cloves garlic, minced
- 1 teaspoon ground cumin
- 1 teaspoon ground turmeric
- 1/2 teaspoon paprika
- 4 cups vegetable broth
- 1 (14.5 oz) can chopped tomatoes
- 2 cups fresh spinach leaves
- Toss with salt and pepper.
- Fresh parsley for garnish (optional)

**Method of Preparation:**

1.  In a big skillet, heat the oil from the olives over a medium-high flame. Add chopped onion, carrots, and celery, and simmer until softened approximately 5 minutes.

2.  Add minced garlic, ground cumin, ground turmeric, and paprika to the saucepan. Cook for another 1-2 minutes, until fragrant.

3.  Add dry green lentils, vegetable broth, and chopped tomatoes (with their liquids) to the saucepan. Bring to a boil, then decrease heat and simmer for 20-25 minutes, until lentils are cooked.

4.  Stir in fresh spinach leaves and simmer for 2-3 minutes, until wilted.

5.  Season the lentil soup with salt and pepper to taste.

6. Ladle the soup into bowls, sprinkle with fresh parsley if preferred, and serve warm.

**Quinoa and Black Bean Stuffed Bell Peppers**

These colorful bell peppers are packed with protein-rich quinoa, black beans, and a variety of aromatic spices, making them a healthy and enjoyable lunch or supper alternative.

Preparation Time: 15 minutes

Cooking Time: 30 minutes

Total Time: 45 minutes

Serving Size: 4

**Ingredients:**

- 4 bell peppers (any color), divided and seeds eliminated
- 1 cup quinoa, cleaned
- 2 cups vegetable broth
- 1 tablespoon olive oil
- 1 onion, diced

- 2 cloves garlic, minced

- 1 teaspoon ground cumin

- 1 teaspoon chilli powder

- 1 (15 ounces) package of black beans, washed and drained

- 1 cup corn kernels (fresh or frozen)

- 1/4 cup chopped fresh cilantro

- Toss with salt and pepper.

- Shredded cheese for topping (optional)

**Method of Preparation:**

1. Preheat the oven to 375°F (190°C). Place the halved bell peppers in a baking tray and set aside.

2. In a saucepan, mix quinoa and vegetable broth. Bring to a boil, then decrease heat and simmer for 15-20 minutes, until quinoa is cooked and liquid is absorbed.

3. In a big pan, heat the olive oil over a moderate flame. Add chopped onion and simmer until softened approximately 5 minutes.

4. Add minced garlic, ground cumin, and chili powder to the skillet. Cook for another 1-2 minutes, until fragrant.

5. Stir in cooked quinoa, black beans, corn kernels, and chopped cilantro. Serve with salt and pepper as needed.

6. Spoon the quinoa and black bean mixture equally into the halved bell peppers.

7. Cover the baking dish with foil and bake in the preheated oven for 25-30 minutes, until the bell peppers are soft.

8. If using shredded cheese, sprinkle it over the filled bell peppers during the final 5 minutes of baking.

9. eliminate from the heat and let cool gently before serving.

**Chicken and Vegetable Stir-Fry with Brown Rice**

This tasty stir-fry is laden with succulent chicken breast, crisp veggies, and aromatic brown rice, making it a nutritious and enjoyable dish for lunch or supper.

Preparation Time: 15 minutes

Cooking Time: 15 minutes

Total Time: 30 minutes

Serving Size: 4

**Ingredients:**

- 1 cup brown rice
- 2 cups water
- 2 teaspoons soy sauce
- 1 tablespoon hoisin sauce
- 1 tablespoon rice vinegar

- 1 teaspoon sesame oil

- 1 tablespoon olive oil

- 1 pound boneless, devoid of skin chicken breast, sliced finely

- 2 cups broccoli florets

- 1 red bell pepper, sliced

- 1 carrot, finely sliced

- 2 cloves garlic, minced

- 1 teaspoon grated ginger

- Toss with salt and pepper.

- Sesame seeds and sliced green onions for garnish (optional)

**Method of Preparation:**

1. In a saucepan, mix brown rice and water. Bring to a boil, then decrease heat and simmer for 40-45 minutes, until rice is soft and water is absorbed.

2. In a small bowl, mix soy sauce, hoisin sauce, rice vinegar, and sesame oil to form the sauce. Set aside.

3. Heat olive oil in a large pan or wok over medium-high heat. Add thinly sliced chicken breast and simmer for 5-7 minutes, until cooked through.

4. Add broccoli florets, sliced red bell pepper, and thinly sliced carrot to the pan. Cook for a further 3-4 minutes, until veggies are crisp-tender.

5. Stir in minced garlic and grated ginger, and simmer for 1-2 minutes, until aromatic.

6. Spread the sauce atop the chicken and veggies in the pan. Stir to coat evenly and simmer for 1-2 minutes, until cooked through.

7. Dish the chicken and vegetable stir-fry over fried brown rice.

8. Sprinkle with sesame seeds and sliced onions that are green, if preferred, and serve hot.

# CHAPTER FIVE

**Satisfying Dinner Options**

**Baked Lemon Herb Chicken with Asparagus**

Tender and flavorful chicken breasts marinated in lemon and herbs served with fresh asparagus for a wholesome and pleasurable evening.

Preparation Time: 10 minutes

Cooking Time: 25 minutes

Total Time: 35 minutes

Serving Size: 2

**Ingredients:**

- 2 boneless, skinless chicken breasts
- 2 tablespoons olive oil
- 2 teaspoons lemon juice
- 2 cloves garlic, minced
- 1 teaspoon dried thyme
- 1 teaspoon dried rosemary
- Salt and pepper to taste

- 1 bunch asparagus, trimmed Lemon slices for garnish (optional)

**Method of Preparation:**

1. Preheat the oven to 400°F (200°C). Prepare a baking dish with a drizzle of olive oil or non-stick spray.

2. In a small bowl, whisk together olive oil, lemon juice, minced garlic, dried thyme, dried rosemary, salt, and pepper to prepare the marinade.

3. Place chicken breasts in the prepared baking dish. Pour the marinade over the chicken and toss to coat evenly.

4. Arrange trimmed asparagus spears around the chicken breasts in the baking dish.

5. Bake in the preheated oven for 20-25 minutes, until the chicken is cooked through and the asparagus is tender.

6. Remove from the oven and let settle for a few minutes before serving.

7. Garnish with lemon slices, if wanted, and serve warm.

**Grilled Shrimp and Vegetable Skewers**

These scrumptious shrimp and vegetable skewers are marinated in a spicy herb and garlic marinade, and then grilled to perfection for a pleasant and healthy dinner option.

Preparation Time: 15 minutes

Cooking Time: 10 minutes

Total Time: 25 minutes

Serving Size: 2

**Ingredients:**

- 1/2 pound huge shrimp, peeled and deveined
- 1 zucchini, sliced into rounds
- 1 yellow bell pepper, sliced into bits
- 1 red onion, chopped into pieces

- 1 tablespoon olive oil

- 2 cloves garlic, minced

- 1 teaspoon dried oregano

- 1 teaspoon dried basil

- Salt and pepper to taste

- Lemon wedges for serving

**Method of Preparation:**

1. When using wooden skewers, get them in water for a minimum of 30 minutes to save them from burning on the grill.

2. In a bowl, add olive oil, minced garlic, dried oregano, dried basil, salt, and pepper to make the marinade.

3. Thread shrimp, zucchini slices, yellow bell pepper pieces, and red onion chunks onto skewers, alternating between the components.

4.  Brush the skewers with the herb and garlic marinade, being sure to cover them evenly.

5.  Preheat the grill to medium-high heat. Grill the skewers for 2-3 minutes on each side, until the shrimp is pink and opaque and the vegetables are cooked and softly browned.

6.  Remove off the grill and transfer the skewers to a serving platter.

7.  Serve the grilled shrimp and vegetable skewers with lemon wedges for squeezing over the top.

## Stuffed Portobello Mushrooms with Spinach and Feta

These robust portobello mushrooms are packed with a tasty combination of spinach, garlic, onions, and feta cheese, then roasted until brown and bubbling for a great vegetarian dinner option.

Preparation Time: 15 minutes

Cooking Time: 25 minutes

Total Time: 40 minutes

Serving Size: 2

**Ingredients:**

- 4 huge portobello mushrooms, stems removed
- 2 tablespoons olive oil
- 2 cloves garlic, minced
- 1/2 onion, finely chopped
- 2 cups fresh spinach leaves

- 1/4 cup crumbled feta cheese

- Salt and pepper to taste

- Fresh parsley for garnish (optional)

**Method of Preparation:**

1. Preheat the oven to 375°F (190°C). Line a baking sheet with parchment paper.

2. Place portobello mushrooms on the prepared baking sheet, gill-side up.

3. In a pan, warm olive oil over moderately high heat. Add minced garlic and chopped onion, and cook until softened about 5 minutes.

4. Add fresh spinach leaves to the skillet and boil until wilted. Remove from heat.

5. Stir in crumbled feta cheese and season with salt and pepper to taste.

6. Spoon the spinach and feta mixture evenly into the cavity of each portobello mushroom.

7. Bake in the preheated oven for 20-25 minutes, until the mushrooms are tender and the mixture is golden and bubbling.

8. remove from your oven and let cool for several minutes before serving.

9. Garnish with fresh parsley, if wanted, and serve warm.

**Cauliflower Rice Stir-Fry with Tofu**

This wonderful stir-fry includes cauliflower rice, tofu, and a variety of colorful vegetables, all blended in a savory soy sauce-based sauce for a terrific and wholesome dinner option.

Preparation Time: 15 minutes

Cooking Time: 15 minutes

Total Time: 30 minutes

Serving Size: 2

**Ingredients:**

- 1 (14 oz) block hard tofu, rinsed and crushed
- 1 tablespoon soy sauce
- 1 tablespoon cornstarch
- 1 tablespoon sesame oil
- 2 cups cauliflower rice
- 1 carrot, thinly sliced
- 1 red bell pepper, thinly sliced
- 1 cup broccoli florets
- 2 cloves garlic, minced
- 2 green onions, sliced
- 2 teaspoons soy sauce
- 1 tablespoon hoisin sauce
- 1 tablespoon rice vinegar
- 1 teaspoon sriracha (optional)
- Sesame seeds for garnish (optional)

**Method of Preparation:**

1. Preheat the oven to 400°F (200°C). Line a baking sheet with parchment paper.

2. Cut the squeezed tofu into cubes and lay them on the prepared baking sheet. Drizzle with soy sauce and sprinkle with cornstarch, tossing to coat evenly.

3. Bake the tofu in the preheated oven for 25-30 minutes, until golden and crispy.

4. Meanwhile, heat sesame oil in a big skillet or wok over medium-high heat. Add cauliflower rice, thinly sliced carrot, thinly sliced red bell pepper, and broccoli florets to the pan. Heat for 5-7 minutes, till vegetables are tender-crisp.

5. Add minced garlic and sliced green onions to the pan, and sauté for an additional 1-2 minutes, until fragrant.

6. In a small bowl, whisk together soy sauce, hoisin sauce, rice vinegar, and sriracha (if using) to make the sauce.

7. Add cooked tofu pieces and sauce to the skillet with the cauliflower rice and vegetables. Toss to coat evenly and heat for 2-3 minutes, until cooked through.

8. Serve the cauliflower rice stir-fry hot, sprinkled with sesame seeds if wanted.

**Turkey Meatballs with Zucchini Noodles**

These scrumptious turkey meatballs are served over spiralized zucchini noodles and coated with a marinara sauce for a healthy and full-dinner alternative.

Preparation Time: 15 minutes

Cooking Time: 25 minutes

Total Time: 40 minutes

Serving Size: 2

**Ingredients:**

- 1 pound ground turkey
- 1/4 cup breadcrumbs
- 1/4 cup grated Parmesan cheese
- 1 egg
- 2 cloves garlic, minced
- 1 tablespoon chopped fresh parsley
- Salt and pepper to taste
- 2 tablespoons olive oil
- 2 zucchini, spiralized into noodles
- 1 cup marinara sauce
- Fresh basil for garnish (optional)

**Method of Preparation:**

1. In a bowl, combine ground turkey, breadcrumbs, grated Parmesan cheese, egg, minced garlic, chopped fresh parsley, salt, and pepper. Mix until thoroughly mixed.

2. Shape the turkey mixture into meatballs, about 1 inch in diameter.

3. Heat olive oil in a large pan over medium heat. Add the turkey meatballs to the pan and cook for 4-5 minutes on each side, until browned and cooked through.

4. While the meatballs are cooking, spiralize the zucchini into noodles using a spiralizer.

5. Once the meatballs are done, remove them from the pan and put aside.

6. In the same skillet, add spiralized zucchini pasta and a marinara sauce. Cook for 2-3 minutes, until the noodles are soft and cooked fully.

7. Return the cooked turkey meatballs to the pan with the zucchini noodles and marinara sauce. Toss to coat evenly.

8. Serve the turkey meatballs and zucchini noodles hot, garnished with fresh basil if liked.

# CHAPTER SIX

**Side Dishes and Salads**

**Garlic Roasted Brussels Sprouts**

These roasted Brussels sprouts are coated in olive oil and garlic and then roasted till golden and crispy for a tasty and healthful side dish.

Preparation Time: 10 minutes

Cooking Time: 25 minutes

Total Time: 35 minutes

Serving Size: 4

**Ingredients:**

- 1 pound Brussels sprouts, trimmed and halved
- 2 tablespoons olive oil
- 4 cloves garlic, minced
- Salt and pepper to taste

**Method of Preparation:**

1. Preheat the oven to 400°F (200°C). Line a baking sheet with parchment paper.

2. In a bowl, mix halved Brussels sprouts with olive oil, minced garlic, salt, and pepper until equally coated.

3. Distribute the Brussels sprouts in one layer on the baking sheet that has been greased.

4. Roast in the preheated oven for 20-25 minutes, stirring halfway through, until the Brussels sprouts are golden and crispy.

5. Remove from the oven and serve hot.

## Lemon Garlic Roasted Asparagus

This easy side dish combines crisp asparagus stalks grilled with lemon and garlic for a burst of flavor and a nutritional complement to any meal.

Preparation Time: 5 minutes

Cooking Time: 15 minutes

Total Time: 20 minutes

Serving Size: 4

**Ingredients:**

- 1 lb asparagus spears, trimmed
- 2 tablespoons olive oil
- 2 cloves garlic, diced Zest of 1 lemon
- Salt and pepper to taste
- Lemon wedges for serving

**Method of Preparation**:

1. Preheat the oven to 400°F (200°C). Line a baking sheet with parchment paper.
2. Place trimmed asparagus spears on the prepared baking sheet.

3. In a small bowl, mix olive oil, minced garlic, lemon zest, salt, and pepper.

4. Drizzle the olive oil mixture over the asparagus spears and toss to coat evenly.

5. Roast in the preheated oven for 12-15 minutes, until the asparagus is tender and gently browned.

6. Remove from the oven and serve hot with lemon wedges for squeezing over the top.

**Quinoa Pilaf with Mixed Vegetables**

This savory quinoa pilaf is filled with various veggies and fragrant herbs, making it a healthful and delightful side dish for any dinner.

Preparation Time: 10 minutes

Cooking Time: 20 minutes

Total Time: 30 minutes

Serving Size: 4

**Ingredients:**

- 1 cup quinoa, washed
- 2 cups vegetable broth 1 tablespoon olive oil
- 1/2 onion, diced
- 2 cloves garlic, minced
- 1 carrot, diced
- 1 bell pepper, diced
- 1 cup frozen peas
- 1 teaspoon dried thyme
- 1 teaspoon dried oregano
- Salt and pepper to taste
- Fresh parsley for garnish (optional)

**Method of Preparation:**

1. In a saucepan, mix quinoa and vegetable broth. Bring to a boil, then decrease heat and simmer for 15-20 minutes, until quinoa is cooked and liquid is absorbed.

2. At this point, heat olive oil in a large pan over medium heat. Add chopped onion and simmer until softened approximately 5 minutes.

3. Add minced garlic, chopped carrot, diced bell pepper, frozen peas, dried thyme, and dried oregano to the skillet. Cook for a further 5-7 minutes, until the veggies are soft.

4. Once the quinoa is done, add it to the pan with the sautéed veggies. Stir to mix.

5. Season the quinoa pilaf with salt and pepper to taste.

6. Garnish with fresh parsley, if preferred, and serve hot.

**Garlic Mashed Cauliflower**

This creamy and savory mashed cauliflower is a low-carb alternative to typical mashed potatoes, making it a nutritious and tasty side dish for any dinner.

Preparation Time: 10 minutes

Cooking Time: 15 minutes

Total Time: 25 minutes

Serving Size: 4

**Ingredients:**

- 1 full head cauliflower, sliced into florets
- 2 cloves garlic, minced
- 2 tablespoons butter or olive oil
- 1/4 cup grated Parmesan cheese
- Salt and pepper to taste
- Chopped chives for garnish (optional)

**Method of Preparation**:

1. Place cauliflower florets in a steamer basket placed over a saucepan of boiling water. Cover and steam for 10-12 minutes, until cauliflower is very soft.

2. Meanwhile, heat butter or olive oil in a small pan over medium heat. Add minced garlic and simmer for 1-2 minutes, until fragrant.

3. Move boiled cauliflower to a food processor or mixer. Add cooked garlic and butter (or olive oil), grated Parmesan cheese, salt, and pepper.

4. Blend until smooth and creamy, scraping down the edges of the bowl as required.

5. Taste and adjust seasoning as required.

6. Transfer mashed cauliflower to a serving dish, sprinkle with chopped chives if preferred, and serve hot.

**Roasted Sweet Potatoes with Maple Cinnamon Glaze**

These soft roasted sweet potatoes are covered in a sweet and aromatic maple cinnamon sauce, making them a wonderful and healthful side dish for any dinner.

Preparation Time: 10 minutes

Cooking Time: 30 minutes

Total Time: 40 minutes

Serving Size: 4

**Ingredients:**

- 2 big sweet potatoes, skinned and cut into pieces
- 2 tablespoons olive oil
- 2 tablespoons maple syrup
- 1 teaspoon ground cinnamon
- Salt to taste
- Chopped pecans for garnish (optional)

**Method of Preparation:**

- Preheat the oven to 400°F (200°C). Line a sheet of baking parchment with paper parchment.

- In a bowl, mix sweet potato cubes with olive oil, maple syrup, ground cinnamon, and salt until equally covered.

- Spread the sweet potato cubes in a single layer on the prepared baking sheet.

- Roast in the preheated oven for 25-30 minutes, stirring halfway through, until the sweet potatoes are soft and caramelized.

- Transfer from the hot oven and transfer to a serving plate.

- Garnish with chopped pecans, if preferred, and serve hot.

# CHAPTER SEVEN

**Smoothies To Revitalize Your Senses**

**Berry Blast Smoothie**

This vivid smoothie is brimming with the benefits of mixed berries, banana, and spinach, making it a refreshing and healthy treat that's excellent for breakfast or a lunchtime snack.

Preparation Time: 5 minutes

Total Time: 5 minutes

Serving Size: 2

**Ingredients:**

- 1 cup mixed berries (strawberries, blueberries, raspberries)
- 1 ripe banana
- 1 cup fresh spinach leaves
- 1/2 cup Greek yogurt
- 1/2 cup almond-based milk (or whatever milk of choice)

- 1 tablespoon honey (optional)
- Ice cubes (optional)

**Method of Preparation:**

1. Place mixed berries, ripe bananas, fresh spinach leaves, Greek yogurt, almond milk, and honey (if using) in a blender.

2. Blend until smooth and creamy, adding ice cubes if required for a cooler smoothie.

3. Pour into glasses and serve immediately.

**Tropical Paradise Smoothie**

Escape to the tropics with this delightful smoothie with pineapple, mango, banana, and coconut milk, blended for a taste of paradise in every drink.

Preparation Time: 5 minutes

Total Time: 5 minutes

Serving Size: 2

**Ingredients:**

- 1 cup pineapple chunks
- 1 cup mango chunks
- 1 ripe banana
- 1/2 cup coconut milk
- 1/2 cup Greek yogurt
- Ice cubes (optional)

**Method of Preparation:**

- In a blender, add pineapple pieces, mango chunks, ripe bananas, coconut milk, and Greek yogurt.
- Blend until smooth and creamy.
- Add ice cubes if required for a cooler smoothie and mix again.
- Pour into glasses and serve immediately.

**Green Goddess Smoothie**

Packed with nutrient-rich greens like spinach and kale, along with creamy avocado and sweet banana, this smoothie is a powerhouse of vitamins and minerals to feed your body and improve your energy levels.

Preparation Time: 5 minutes

Total Time: 5 minutes

Serving Size: 2

**Ingredients:**

- 1 cup fresh spinach leaves
- 1 cup kale leaves, stems removed
- 1 ripe banana
- 1/2 avocado
- 1 cup coconut water (or any drink of choice)
- Juice of 1/2 lime
- Ice cubes (optional)

**Method of Preparation:**

1. Place fresh spinach leaves, kale leaves, ripe banana, avocado, coconut water, and lime juice in a blender.

2. Blend until smooth and creamy.

3. Add ice cubes if required for a cooler smoothie and mix again.

4. Pour into glasses and serve immediately.

**Banana Berry Protein Smoothie**

This protein-packed smoothie mixes the sweetness of banana and berries with the punch of protein powder, making it a great post-workout refill or a satisfying breakfast alternative.

Preparation Time: 5 minutes

Total Time: 5 minutes

Serving Size: 2

**Ingredients:**

- 1 ripe banana
- 1 cup mixed berries (strawberries, blueberries, raspberries)
- 1 scoop vanilla protein powder
- 1 cup almond milk (or other milk of choice)
- Ice cubes (optional)

**Method of Preparation:**

- In a blender, add ripe banana, mixed berries, vanilla protein powder, and almond milk.
- Blend until smooth and creamy.
- Add ice cubes if required for a cooler smoothie and mix again.
- Pour into glasses and serve immediately.

**Creamy Coconut Mango Smoothie**

Transport yourself to a tropical paradise with this lusciously creamy smoothie combining juicy mango, coconut milk, and a dash of vanilla, producing a refreshing and decadent delight.

Preparation Time: 5 minutes

Total Time: 5 minutes

Serving Size: 2

**Ingredients:**

- 1 ripe mango, peeled and sliced
- 1/2 cup coconut milk
- 1/2 cup Greek yogurt
- 1 tablespoon honey (optional)
- 1/2 teaspoon vanilla extract
- Ice cubes (optional)

**Method of Preparation:**

- In a blender, add chopped ripe mango, coconut milk, Greek yogurt, honey (if using), and vanilla extract.
- Blend until smooth and creamy.
- Add ice cubes if required for a cooler smoothie and mix again.
- Pour into glasses and serve immediately.

# CHAPTER EIGHT

**Sweet Treats for Sensory Delight**

**Avocado Chocolate Mousse**

Indulge in this rich and creamy chocolate mousse prepared with avocado for a healthy twist. It's luscious, silky, and delicious, great for quenching your sweet desires.

Preparation Time: 10 minutes

Chilling Time: 1 hour

Total Time: 1 hour 10 minutes

Serving Size: 2

**Ingredients:**

- 1 ripe avocado
- 1/4 cup cocoa powder
- 1/4 cup maple syrup or honey
- 1 teaspoon vanilla extract
- Pinch of salt
- Fresh berries for garnish (optional)

**Method of Preparation:**

1. Scoop the flesh of the ripe avocado into a blender or food processor.

2. Add cocoa powder, maple syrup or honey, vanilla essence, and a bit of salt to the blender.

3. Blend until smooth and creamy, scraping down the sides as required.

4. Transfer the chocolate mousse to serving plates or ramekins.

5. Cover and refrigerate for at least 1 hour to cool and solidify.

6. Serve the dish chilled, sprinkled with freshly picked fruit if desired.

**Banana Oatmeal Cookies**

These soft and chewy cookies are prepared with ripe bananas, oats, and a hint of cinnamon for natural sweetness and warmth. They're nutritious, soothing, and excellent for a guilt-free treat.

Preparation Time: 10 minutes

Baking Time: 12-15 minutes

Total Time: 25 minutes

Serving Size: Makes 12 cookies

**Ingredients:**

- 2 ripe bananas, mashed
- 1 cup rolled oats
- 1/4 cup raisins or chocolate chips (optional)
- 1/2 teaspoon ground cinnamon
- Pinch of salt

- 1/4 cup diced nuts (such as hazelnuts or pecans) (optional)

**Method of Preparation:**

1. Preheat the oven to 350°F (175°C). Line a baking sheet with parchment paper.

2. In a mixing dish, add mashed ripe bananas, rolled oats, raisins, or chocolate chips (if used), ground cinnamon, a touch of salt, and chopped nuts (if using). Mix until completely blended.

3. Drop spoonfuls of the cookie dough onto the prepared baking sheet, spacing them apart.

4. Flatten each cookie gently with the back of a spoon or your fingertips.

5. Bake in the preheated oven for 12-15 minutes, until the cookies are golden brown and firm.

6. Remove from the oven and allow to rest on the baking sheet for a few minutes before moving to a wire rack to cool fully.

**Apple Cinnamon Baked Oatmeal Cups**

These individual-sized baked oatmeal cups are flavored with fresh apples, toasty cinnamon, and a dash of maple syrup. They're healthy, portable, and excellent for a quick breakfast or snack on the run.

Preparation Time: 10 minutes

Baking Time: 25 minutes

Total Time: 35 minutes

Serving Size: Makes 12 oatmeal cups

**Ingredients:**

- 2 cups rolled oats
- 1 teaspoon baking powder
- 1 teaspoon ground cinnamon
- Pinch of salt

- 1 1/2 cups milk made from almonds (or other milk of preference)
- 1/4 cup maple syrup
- 1 big egg
- 1 teaspoon vanilla extract
- 1 apple, peeled, cored, and diced
- Chopped nuts for garnish (optional)

**Method of Preparation:**

1. Preheat the oven to 350°F (175°C). Grease a muffin tray or line it with silicone muffin liners.

2. In a mixing dish, add rolled oats, baking powder, powdered cinnamon, and a sprinkle of salt.

3. In a separate dish, mix almond milk, maple syrup, egg, and vanilla extract until completely incorporated.

4. Pour the wet ingredients into the dry ingredients and stir until thoroughly combined.

5. Fold in chopped apple until equally distributed throughout the batter.

6. Divide the oatmeal mixture equally among the muffin cups, filling each approximately 3/4 full.

7. Sprinkle chopped nuts on top of each oatmeal cup, if using.

8. Bake in the preheated oven for 25 minutes, or until the oatmeal cups are firm and golden brown on top.

9. Remove from the oven and allow to cool in the muffin tray for a few minutes before transferring to a wire rack to cool fully.

**Lemon Blueberry Muffins**

These soft and tasty muffins are filled with luscious blueberries and zesty lemon flavor. They're light, moist, and excellent for a pleasant breakfast or snack.

Preparation Time: 15 minutes

Baking Time: 20-25 minutes

Total Time: 40 minutes

Serving Size: Makes 12 muffins

**Ingredients:**

- 2 cups all-purpose flour
- 1/2 cup granulated sugar
- 2 tablespoons baking powder
- 1/2 teaspoon baking soda
- Pinch of salt
- 1 cup Greek yogurt
- 1/4 cup dissolved coconut milk or unsalted butter

- 2 big eggs

- Zest of 1 lemon

- 2 teaspoons fresh lemon juice

- 1 teaspoon vanilla extract

- 1 1/2 cups fresh or frozen blueberries

**Method of Preparation:**

1. Preheat the oven to 375°F (190°C). Assemble a muffin tray with liners made of paper.

2. In a large mixing basin, whisk together all-purpose flour, granulated sugar, baking powder, baking soda, and a sprinkle of salt.

3. In another dish, mix Greek yogurt, melted coconut oil or unsalted butter, eggs, lemon zest, lemon juice, and vanilla essence until smooth.

4. Pour the wet ingredients into the dry ingredients and stir until barely mixed.

5. Gently fold in the blueberries until equally distributed throughout the batter.

6. Divide the mixture equally among the prepared muffin cups, filling each approximately 3/4 full.

7. Bake in the preheated oven for 20-25 minutes, or until the muffins are golden brown and a toothpick inserted into the middle comes out clean.

8. Remove from the oven and allow to cool in the muffin tray for a few minutes before transferring to a wire rack to cool fully.

**Coconut Flour Banana Bread**

This moist and tasty banana bread is baked with coconut flour for a gluten-free and grain-free twist. It's naturally sweetened with ripe bananas and excellent for breakfast or a snack.

Preparation Time: 15 minutes

Baking Time: 50-55 minutes

Total Time: 1 hour 10 minutes

Serving Size: Makes 1 loaf (approximately 10 slices)

**Ingredients:**

- 4 ripe bananas, mashed
- 4 big eggs
- 1/4 cup melted coconut oil
- 1/4 cup maple syrup or honey
- 1 teaspoon vanilla extract
- 3/4 cup coconut flour
- 1 teaspoon baking soda
- 1/2 teaspoon ground cinnamon
- Pinch of salt
- Chopped nuts for topping (optional)

**Method of Preparation:**

1. Preheat the oven to 350°F (175°C). Grease a 9x5-inch loaf pan or line it with parchment paper.

2. In a large mixing bowl, whisk together mashed ripe bananas, eggs, melted coconut oil, maple syrup or honey, and vanilla extract until thoroughly blended.

3. In another dish, whisk together coconut flour, baking soda, ground cinnamon, and a sprinkle of salt.

4. Gradually add the dry ingredients to the liquid components, stirring until no lumps remain and a homogeneous batter develops.

5. Pour the batter into the prepared loaf pan, smoothing the surface with a spatula.

6. Sprinkle chopped nuts on top of the batter, if using.

7. Bake in the preheated oven for 50-55 minutes, or until the top is golden brown and a toothpick inserted into the middle comes out clean.

8. Remove from the oven and allow rest in the loaf pan for 10 minutes before transferring to a wire rack to cool fully.

# CHAPTER NINE

## Tips for Efficient Meal Planning Batch Cooking Strategies for Busy Days, Quick and Easy Meal Prep Recipes

In the rush and bustle of contemporary life, finding time to make healthful meals may seem like a difficult task—especially while negotiating the obstacles of treating peripheral neuropathy. But worry not, because, with a little organization and imagination, you can expedite your meal preparation process, ensuring that healthful meals are always within reach. Let's examine some suggestions for effective meal planning, batch cooking tactics for busy days, and fast and simple meal prep recipes to fuel your path toward nerve health and energy.

**Tips for Efficient Meal Planning:**

**Set Aside Time for Planning:** Dedicate a certain day each week to meal planning and grocery shopping. Use this time to explore recipes, prepare a meal plan for the week ahead, and build a shopping list of goods you'll need.

**Keep it Simple:** Focus on meals that need little materials and preparation time. Look for dishes that can be done in one pot or pan, such as stir-fries, sheet pan dinners, or slow cooker meals, to simplify your cooking process.

**Embrace Versatility:** Choose items that can be utilized in numerous meals throughout the week. For example, if you roast a batch of veggies on Sunday, you may use them as a side dish, add them to salads, or integrate them into grain bowls throughout the week.

**Prep Ahead:** Take advantage of downtime throughout the week to prep items in advance. Wash and cut veggies, marinade meats, and prepare grains or legumes ahead of time to save time on hectic weekdays.

**Batch Cooking Strategies for Busy Days:**

**Choose Batch-Friendly dishes:** Opt for dishes that lend themselves well to batch cooking, such as soups, stews, casseroles, and grain-based salads. These meals frequently enhance in taste when cooked ahead of time and maybe portioned out for convenient reheating throughout the week.

**Invest in Storage Containers:** Stock up on a range of airtight containers in varying sizes to keep batch-cooked meals and supplies. Mason jars, glass containers, and silicone storage bags are wonderful alternatives for keeping food fresh and organized in the fridge or freezer.

**mark and Date**: To minimize confusion and food waste, mark your storage containers with the name of the meal and the date it was produced. This makes it simple to get a meal from the fridge or freezer and guarantees that nothing is lost or forgotten.

**Freeze Extras:** If you find yourself with leftover batch-cooked meals, don't hesitate to freeze them for future use. Soups, stews, and casseroles may be portioned up into individual portions and frozen for fast and handy dinners on busy days.

**Quick and Easy Meal Prep Recipes:**
**Overnight Oats:** Combine rolled oats, milk or plant-based milk, Greek yogurt, and your favorite toppings (such as berries, nuts, seeds, or nut butter) in a jar or container. Refrigerate

overnight, and have a tasty and healthy breakfast ready to go in the morning.

**Mason Jar Salads**: Layer salad ingredients in a mason jar, beginning with dressing at the bottom and finishing with leafy greens on top. When ready to dine, just shake the jar to spread the dressing evenly and enjoy a fresh and tasty salad on the move.

**Sheet Pan Dinners:** Toss chopped veggies and protein of your choice (such as chicken, tofu, or fish) with olive oil and spices on a sheet pan. Roast in the oven until cooked through, then serve with cooked grains or a side salad for an easy and comforting supper.

**Veggie Stir-Fry:** Heat oil in a pan or wok, then stir-fry your favorite veggies until tender-crisp. Add cooked protein (such as shrimp, tofu, or tempeh) and your favorite sauce, and serve overcooked rice or noodles for a fast and tasty stir-fry supper.

With these tactics, methods, and recipes in your culinary arsenal, you'll be well-equipped to manage meal planning and preparation with ease—even on the busiest of days. By spending a little time and working early, you'll guarantee that nutritional meals are constantly at your fingertips, supporting your path toward nerve health and vitality. So, let's embrace the art of efficient meal planning, bulk cooking, and meal prep, and appreciate the tastes of health and well-being with every mouthful.

**The 14 Days Meal Plan**

**Day 1:**

Breakfast: Warm Quinoa Breakfast Bowl

Lunch: Grilled Salmon Salad with Avocado

Dinner: Baked Lemon Herb Chicken with Asparagus

Snack: Almond Butter and Banana Rice Cakes

**Day 2:**

Breakfast: Banana Nut Oatmeal

Lunch: Turkey and Veggie Wrap with Hummus

Dinner: Grilled Shrimp and Vegetable Skewers

Snack: Trail Mix with Nuts and Dried Fruit

**Day 3:**

Breakfast: Avocado Toast with Poached Egg

Lunch: Lentil Soup with Spinach and Tomatoes

Dinner: Stuffed Portobello Mushrooms with Spinach and Feta

Snack: Roasted Chickpeas with Spices

**Day 4:**

Breakfast: Berry Smoothie Bowl

Lunch: Quinoa and Black Bean Stuffed Bell Peppers

Dinner: Cauliflower Rice stir-fried with Tofu

Snack: Veggie Sticks with Hummus

**Day 5:**

Breakfast: Spinach and Mushroom Frittata

Lunch: Chicken and Vegetable Stir-Fry with Brown Rice

Dinner: Turkey Meatballs with Zucchini Noodles

Snack: Greek Yogurt with Honey and Almonds

**Day 6:**

Breakfast: Warm Quinoa Breakfast Bowl

Lunch: Grilled Salmon Salad with Avocado

Dinner: Baked Lemon Herb Chicken with Asparagus

Snack: Almond Butter and Banana Rice Cakes

**Day 7:**

Breakfast: Banana Nut Oatmeal

Lunch: Turkey and Veggie Wrap with Hummus

Dinner: Grilled Shrimp and Vegetable Skewers

Snack: Trail Mix with Nuts and Dried Fruit

**Day 8:**

Breakfast: Avocado Toast with Poached Egg

Lunch: Lentil Soup with Spinach and Tomatoes

Dinner: Stuffed Portobello Mushrooms with Spinach and Feta

Snack: Roasted Chickpeas with Spices

**Day 9:**

Breakfast: Berry Smoothie Bowl

Lunch: Quinoa and Black Bean Stuffed Bell Peppers

Dinner: Cauliflower Rice stir-fried with Tofu

Snack: Veggie Sticks with Hummus

**Day 10:**

Breakfast: Spinach and Mushroom Frittata

Lunch: Chicken and Vegetable Stir-Fry with Brown Rice

Dinner: Turkey Meatballs with Zucchini Noodles

Snack: Greek Yogurt with Honey and Almonds

**Day 11:**

Breakfast: Warm Quinoa Breakfast Bowl

Lunch: Grilled Salmon Salad with Avocado

Dinner: Baked Lemon Herb Chicken with Asparagus

Snack: Almond Butter and Banana Rice Cakes

**Day 12:**

Breakfast: Banana Nut Oatmeal

Lunch: Turkey and Veggie Wrap with Hummus

Dinner: Grilled Shrimp and Vegetable Skewers

Snack: Trail Mix with Nuts and Dried Fruit

**Day 13**:

Breakfast: Avocado Toast with Poached Egg

Lunch: Lentil Soup with Spinach and Tomatoes

Dinner: Stuffed Portobello Mushrooms with Spinach and Feta

Snack: Roasted Chickpeas with Spices

**Day 14:**

Breakfast: Berry Smoothie Bowl

Lunch: Quinoa and Black Bean Stuffed Bell Peppers

Dinner: Cauliflower Rice stir-fried with Tofu

Snack: Veggie Sticks with Hummus

## CONCLUSION

**Celebrating Your Journey to Better Health**

As you reach the last pages of this cookbook, take a minute to think of the trip you've gone upon—a journey toward improved health, resilience, and vitality in the face of peripheral neuropathy. With each dish you've studied, each ingredient you've relished, and each meal you've cooked, you've made a major step forward on the road to health and well-being.

But this journey isn't just about the food on your plate—it's about the strength that comes from taking charge of your health and embracing the transforming power of nutrition. It's about realizing the significant link between what you eat and how you feel and utilizing that knowledge to feed your body, mind, and soul from the inside.

While you embark on your path, know that you are not alone. Within these pages, you've discovered not just recipes, but a network of support—a tribe of kindred travelers on the neuropathy route, each with their tales, problems, and victories to share. Together, we celebrate your bravery, your perseverance, and your resolve to recover your energy, one delicious meal at a time.

## Resources for Further Exploration

Your quest for nerve health and vigor doesn't stop here. To continue your investigation and enhance your knowledge of peripheral neuropathy therapy with diet, try examining the following resources:

Books and Publications: Dive further into the science of nutrition and neuropathy with books and publications produced by specialists in the subject. Look for works that concentrate on neuropathy care, nutritional methods, and holistic approaches to wellbeing.

Online Communities and Support Groups: Connect with people having similar problems and experiences in online communities and support groups devoted to peripheral neuropathy. Share your story, seek advice and support, and gain from the knowledge of others who have traveled this route before you.

Healthcare Professionals: Consult with your healthcare practitioner or a qualified dietitian for tailored direction and support in controlling peripheral neuropathy via nutrition. They can help you establish a personalized meal plan, manage any dietary issues or limits, and assess your progress over time.

Cooking lessons and Workshops: Expand your culinary abilities and repertoire with cooking lessons and workshops focusing on nerve-friendly dishes and food preparation methods. These hands-on experiences give vital insights and inspiration for implementing good eating habits into your everyday life.

Thank you for permitting us to be part of your experience. May your journey be blessed with richness, vigor, and steadfast conviction in the power of food to heal, nourish, and change. Here's to you, here's to us, and here's to the bright, resilient spirit that drives us ahead, one delicious mouthful at a time.